Diabetes Diet

How to improve, manage, and prevent diabetes with the help of food!

Table Of Contents

Introduction	V
Chapter 1 - Diabetes 101	1
Chapter 2 - Symptoms And Diagnosis	5
Chapter 3 - Getting Started	11
Chapter 4 - All About Nutrition	15
Chapter 5 - What To Avoid	21
Chapter 6 - Meal Tips And Suggestions	27
Chapter 7 - Coping With The Real World	31
Chapter 8 - Additional Advice	39
Conclusion	45

Introduction

I want to thank you and congratulate you for downloading the book, *"Diabetes Diet"*.

This book contains helpful information about diabetes, and how it can be improved with diet and lifestyle changes.

Diabetes affects a large number of people, and its prevalence is increasing at an alarming rate! This book will explain to you the different types of diabetes, their causes, signs and symptoms, and how they are diagnosed.

Diabetes can be a debilitating condition with many negative outcomes. Luckily, it can be controlled greatly with diet, and in many instances improved and reversed.

This book includes tips and techniques to help you manage, and avoid diabetes with the power of diet! You will discover the different foods to avoid, and those to consume. To make it easy to start making dietary changes, this book also includes some sample meal plans to try out!

Thanks again for downloading this book, I hope you enjoy it and find it helpful in managing and improving your diabetes!

Chapter 1 - Diabetes 101

You probably have already heard of diabetes. You may have seen it in the news, social media, or other sources. You may even know co-workers, acquaintances, friends, or relatives who suffer from it. Perhaps you suffer from it yourself. You may also know that diabetes can't be cured and that obese people are prone to developing it. While you are familiar with the disease, you may want to further expand your knowledge on this topic.

Diabetes mellitus, simply known as diabetes, is one of the most widespread diseases in the world. More than 150 million people worldwide suffer from diabetes and this number is projected to double by 2025. Furthermore, the total deaths caused by diabetes are expected to rise by over half within the next ten years and by over 80% in countries with upper-middle income. It isn't surprising that the World Health Organization considers diabetes as an emerging global epidemic. So now you may ask: why is diabetes so deadly?

Diabetes is a chronic illness, also known as a metabolism disorder, wherein a person's blood glucose level is higher than normal. Glucose is a simple sugar that is broken down from food people eat. This supplies energy for the body to execute metabolic processes like muscle development and digestion. Insulin, a hormone produced by the pancreas, enables the body to utilize glucose and regulates it in the bloodstream. It triggers a series of reactions to convert glucose into energy. Someone who is suffering from diabetes has insufficient insulin. In effect, more glucose will remain in their blood system. Unchanged glucose isn't beneficial. Hence, the body will choose to find alternative sources of energy. It may break down fats and protein while releasing glucose through urine. This may damage the organs, nerves, and blood vessels.

Types

There are two types of diabetes. Type 1 diabetes or insulin-dependent diabetes occurs when the pancreas is unable to create insulin. This accounts for 10% of adults suffering from diabetes. Although this can develop at any age, children and those below 40 are prone to being diagnosed with this type. As it is common in children, this type can also be referred to as juvenile diabetes.

Type 2 diabetes, or non-insulin-dependent diabetes, is more common. Although the body may be producing insulin, this isn't being efficiently used. In some cases, the cells within the body will ignore the insulin. This form of diabetes accounts for 90% of diabetes cases around the world. Studies have shown that at least one out of three people will develop type 2 diabetes within their lifetime. While children are diagnosed more often with type 1 diabetes, the recent years have reported more young people being diagnosed with type 2 diabetes.

Modern research has produced interesting findings related to type 2 diabetes. Specifically, young adults whose parents were inflicted with type 2 diabetes were observed. The said group was comprised of thin, healthy people who were free from diabetes during that period. However, researchers noticed that these individuals were more resistant to insulin. If they were given a dose of glucose, the simple sugar would build up in their bodies. Looking at the molecular level, it was found that their muscle cells possessed small amounts of fat. Initially, insulin would be created and sent to the muscles. However, the fats hindered the work of insulin.

Now you may ask why there is fat present in the first place. Generally, muscle cells store a small amount of fat to be used for energy. However, for the observed adults, it was seen that their fat levels were 80% higher than those found in other people. This caused fat buildup that interfered with the interaction of cells to insulin.

While the first two types of diabetes are chronic conditions, the third can be temporary. Gestational diabetes occurs only in 4% of pregnant women. Although this type of diabetes disappears after pregnancy, around 50% of women who experienced this develop type 2 diabetes after several years.

While these are the currently established types of diabetes, studies have suggested a prediabetes phase. This refers to the stage wherein the individual's blood sugar is higher than normal. However, this isn't high enough to qualify the individual to have diabetes. Nonetheless, this indicates a higher risk of developing type 2 diabetes. In the United States, one out of three adults is reported to have prediabetes. However, nine out of ten of those with prediabetes are unaware of their condition.

Causes and Risk Factors

Because diabetes affects millions of people worldwide, your next question may be to ask what causes this disease. While research has pointed out the lack of insulin as the primary culprit, inefficient insulin production is said to be inherited. However, studies on identical twins have discovered that if one twin has type 1 diabetes, the other has a less than 40% chance of acquiring it. Hence, one's environment and exposure to food and infections may be the primary contributors to type 1 diabetes.

On the other hand, studies have shown that type 2 diabetes is significantly affected by one's lifestyle. In fact, overweight people have a much higher risk of developing type 2 diabetes. If one eats unhealthy food and fails to engage in physical activity, their body tends to release chemicals that would destabilize the metabolic systems. This may affect insulin production. Aside from excessive weight, the risk also rises as one ages. People above 45 are more prone to the disease. Although experts are unsure why this happens, they propose that people who age tend to become less physically active and gain more weight.

Ethnicity also indicates a higher risk for type 2 diabetes development. Specifically, those of African, Pacific Island, Middle Eastern, or South Asian descent are more prone to the disease. Finally, men who have low testosterone levels were also reported to have a higher likelihood of developing the disease. Low testosterone may be linked to insulin resistance.

As for prediabetes, no one knows for sure what exactly causes it. Because many people are unaware that they even have the condition, they can just go on with their normal lives until they eventually discover that they have developed diabetes. In cases like these, it is advisable to look at the risk factors related to diabetes and see if you qualify for these.

Chapter 2 - Symptoms and Diagnosis

Perhaps the most important question to answer is 'how do you know if you are experiencing diabetes?' Determining if you are suffering from diabetes is essential to alleviate your condition. Although this can't be cured, you can act as soon as possible to prevent it from worsening.

Symptoms

Glucose is vital for daily bodily processes. Altering the glucose-regulating system will result in chaotic effects. Because of the increased glucose levels within the body, various symptoms would be felt by people experiencing type 1 or 2 diabetes. For one, frequent urination is possible as a high amount of glucose can force fluids out of the cells. These would be delivered to the kidneys for disposal. While urination is a normal process, frequent visits to bathroom may bear negative effects such as dehydration. In effect, you would often feel thirsty. Hence, urinating and needing to drink more would be possible signs of diabetes.

However, high glucose levels can also create more alarming symptoms. Specifically, the body would have difficulty in healing. This would cause sores and cuts to remain for prolonged periods of time. Hence, they would be more prone to infection. Furthermore, although rising blood sugar levels are initially unnoticed, this would spell severe effects in the long run. Foot problems, kidney diseases, heart disease, and other conditions can arise due to the unregulated presence of glucose. Blurred vision might also occur because the high glucose levels can lead to eye lens swelling.

Another major symptom of diabetes is fatigue. In your daily activities, you may quickly feel tired and take a handful of breaks. You may wonder why you feel exhausted after several minutes of light work. Since glucose is broken down to produce energy, the incapacity to utilize this would alter the amount of available energy in the body. Without sufficient energy, your body wouldn't be able to function properly. Hence, you would easily feel tired and would need to recover.

While there are numerous symptoms for diabetes, people who experience prediabetes don't display obvious symptoms. However, you can examine you risk factors, such as age, weight, and lifestyle, to see if you could possibly have the condition. The best way to see if you are suffering from prediabetes involves undergoing lab tests.

Diagnosis

If you are experiencing the symptoms of diabetes, you can proceed to the doctor to get tested. Because the early phase of type 2 diabetes may show no symptoms, drawing blood from the patient would be the primary mode to assess the levels of glucose in the bloodstream.

The most basic test used to diagnose prediabetes and diabetes is the blood test. Here, you would fast for 8-hours prior to the test which would be done in the morning. You shouldn't consume anything within the fasting period to avoid test errors. Afterwards, the doctor would measure the glucose within the patient's blood. If your blood sugar level is 126 mg/dL or higher, the test would be repeated. If the same result is received, the doctor would conclude that the patient may be suffering from diabetes. On the other hand, results that show 100 mg/dL to 125 mg/dL would indicate prediabetes.

The A1C, also known as the HbA1c, hemoglobin A1c, or glycohemoglobin test, can detect prediabetes and type 2 diabetes. However, this wouldn't be recommended to assess the patient for type 1 diabetes or gestational diabetes. Hemoglobin carries oxygen and gives color to red blood cells. The A1C test would measure the amount of glucose that has entered the blood and stuck to the hemoglobin. This is a special blood test that reports your average blood glucose level over the last three months. In effect, it wouldn't show fluctuations that may occur in your daily life. Hence, this test can be more convenient for you because you wouldn't have to fast for several hours before the test. For this test, the result would be indicated by a percentage. If the result reads 5.7 to 6.4%, prediabetes may be indicated. These people would be retested after a year. On the other hand, people with an A1C result above 6.0% would be highly likely to develop diabetes while readings above 6.5% signify the presence of diabetes.

You may also undergo the oral glucose tolerance test to confirm diabetes, gestational diabetes, and prediabetes. In summary, you would consume water with 75g of glucose. After two hours, the doctor would measure the glucose levels in your blood. If the sugar level reads 200 mg/dL or higher, you would be suspected of diabetes.

The random blood sugar test is another possible tool to confirm diabetes. The doctor would measure the glucose levels of your blood at any time within the day. This wouldn't take into account the last time you ate. A reading of 200 mg/dL or higher would indicate diabetes.

Although these tests can be accurate, the results may vary. Since glucose levels fluctuate depending on one's exercise, stress, meals, and other activities, results may not be fully accurate even if you fasted. Also, the tests may produce varying results depending on the sample handling, temperature, and equipment used. In effect, it is best to undergo several tests to see the consistency of the results.

Significance of early diagnosis

If you are at risk of diabetes, you should take the situation seriously. Consult a doctor and begin planning ways to cope with your condition. Even if tests show that you are currently free of the disease, you should prevent it from developing. If left untreated, diabetes will let blood sugar levels continue to rise and lead to complications.

Diabetic retinopathy can lead to visual disability and blindness. Specifically, diabetes can affect the blood vessels within the retina of the eye. This may eventually worsen and cause loss of vision. Diabetes can also trigger more severe problems in the cataract and glaucoma. According to studies, 2% of people who have had diabetes for over 15 years become blind. Ten percent will suffer from being visually handicapped.

Diabetic foot disease is another possible result. Because of the altered state of nerves and blood vessels, blood flow may be less inefficient in parts like the leg. If there are cuts or wounds in these areas, these would slowly heal and infections would be highly likely. In effect, severe cases may call for the amputation of the infected area.

Diabetic neuropathy is another result of the illness. Being the most common complication, diabetic neuropathy affects over half of the people with diabetes. This state causes damage to the limbs and sensory loss. Men may also suffer from impotence.

Kidney failure may also happen due to high levels of glucose. Because of the combined forces of high blood pressure and high blood glucose, renal damage would be more severe.

Finally, perhaps the most problematic complication that can arise is heart disease. According to studies, over half of the deaths of diabetics are results of heart-related problems. They are more prone to heart attacks and strokes. The possibility would be higher if they smoke, drink alcohol, or don't exercise.

Treatment

Even if you may be suffering from diabetes, this doesn't mean your life is over. There are many methods to respond to the sickness so that you can continue living a normal life. Although treatment can range from undergoing extensive therapy sessions, taking medications, or even surgery for complications, the patient can find natural ways to combat the disease. This includes improving your lifestyle and daily habits. Since the disease does involve glucose from food, monitoring your diet is essential to decrease the severity of the illness.

Chapter 3 - Getting Started

If you are a diabetic, you can find ways to control your condition. Since diabetes involves increased sugar levels, you want to lower this. Achieving this state involves eating healthily and staying fit. According to experts, losing even 5% of one's total weight would significantly lower blood sugar and retain it at normal levels. This would lead to lowered cholesterol levels and blood pressure. Simultaneously, you can experience better energy levels and an increased sense of wellbeing.

Knowing Your Body Type

As being overweight is the most significant risk factor for developing diabetes, you would initially want to avoid this state. However, everyone has differing body fat levels. You need to know your body type. If a large amount of body fat is located around your abdomen, you will have a higher chance of developing diabetes compared to those with more fat in their thighs or hips. The first body type refers to the "apple-shaped body" while the latter is called the "pear-shaped body."

People with "apple-shaped bodies" store fats near the liver and other abdominal organs. In effect, insulin resistance would be more likely. This would be more problematic than "pear-shaped" figures who would be more concerned with fatty areas farther away from these sites. Aside from body types, your gender will also play a role in the need for weight loss. Men and women who have waist circumferences above 40 inches and 35 inches, respectively, are more prone to diabetes.

Knowing this, you can measure your waist circumference. By placing a tape measure around your abdomen, you can determine if you are in the risk category or not.

Mentally Preparing Yourself

Once you are familiar with your body, you can proceed to developing meal plans and strategies to cut down your weight. To successfully plan future meals, you should consider the following tips.

1) **Set your goals.**

You have to understand why you must manage your diet. Although your obvious answer would involve wanting to control diabetes, you need to dig deeper. Would you want to control it to live a healthy and long life? Are you doing this to remain healthy for your kids or loved ones? All these questions should be clearly answered for you to maintain the motivation to control and even reverse your diabetes. In setting what you want to achieve, you will remain focused in the long run and continue having the passion to live a better life.

2) **Have a budget**

Preparing healthy food entails preparing the proper ingredients. While cooking food can be exciting, you should also maximize your budget to ensure that the new meal plans won't be a burden on your daily expenses. If you want to try out a certain dish but may find it to be expensive, you can look for alternative ingredients or other great recipes. Remembering that these meal plans will be used every day, you have to create plans that fit your budget and still provide you sufficient nutrition.

3) **Knowledge is power**

You may have the right mindset and goals, but you may not know the right steps to take. Learning is a continuous process that you should embrace throughout your dieting journey. Constantly reading books and other reliable sources may help you discover new healthy recipes, techniques, and other diabetes-related news that would benefit you. If ever you feel lost with your plans, don't be afraid to ask for help. Your dietitian, physician, and other trusted friends can help you and suggest better options. Just make sure to be critical in discerning if these are worth trying out.

4) **Patience is a virtue**

This ageless saying is very applicable to your condition. Knowing that diabetes is a chronic condition, you have to accept that you may have to live with it for the rest of your life unless a cure is discovered. However, as explained in the previous chapter, you shouldn't look at this negatively and feel that your life is over. In patiently following safe and effective diet plans, you can reduce the effects of diabetes and function normally. In some instances, diabetics may even forget that they do have diabetes because their healthy lifestyle has minimized the effects of the disease. Of course, results won't come fast. You will have to dedicate yourself to your plans, no matter what happens.

Chapter 4 - All about Nutrition

Nutrition refers to the process of eating appropriate food that would aid in growth and development. In the case of diabetic patients, nutrition is necessary to manage their diabetes and avoid severe complications. Usually, you will undergo a diabetes diet, also referred to as medical nutrition therapy for diabetes. This isn't a restrictive set of meals. Rather, it ensures that you are following a healthy meal plan that will provide you the nutrients that you need without having to consume high amounts of calories or fats. In reality, a diabetes diet can produce great results for everyone.

Why should I?

If you still feel uneasy about letting go of your former meals for healthier options, you have to remember that your weight and blood sugar are critical for your health. If you eat excessive amounts of fats and calories, your blood glucose can rise and lead to complications. You can experience hyperglycemia in the short-run and chronic problems like heart damage in the long-run. Furthermore, it would be difficult to manage your health if you are overweight. For people with type 2 diabetes, weight loss is crucial to control blood glucose and prevent complications.

There are many myths that revolve around diets. If you want successful results, you need to understand the facts and not rely on gossip. Here are some of the most popular dieting myths and why they're wrong:

1) **Myth: High-protein diets are the best.**

   Truth: Although protein can help build your muscles, eating too much protein can contribute to insulin resistance. Hence, you shouldn't focus only on meat for your future diet. Keeping a balance between proteins, fats, and carbohydrates is essential for the body to function. More of this will be discussed in the latter parts of the chapter.

2) **Myth: You must always cut the carbs.**

   Truth: You don't. Considering a balanced diet, you just have to control the serving sizes and assess the best carbohydrates for your plan. However, it is recommended that you consider whole grains as these provide fiber and keep blood sugar levels lower.

3) **Myth: You will never eat sugar.**

   Truth: You can afford to live with sugar. Moderation is the key to enjoy these food and you just have to properly set these in your schedule. Of course, doing exercise can help you prepare for these sweet delights.

4) **Myth: Diet food tastes bad.**

   Truth: Well, the reality is that there are many recipes and suggestions that are nourishing and delicious. Because these focus on vegetables, fruits, and other healthy food, you can create fine dishes that can satisfy your cravings. You just need to be creative, patient, and determined.

5) Myth: You can only eat special meals for diabetes.

Truth: Diabetic meals can be expensive and may have no advantage over normal meals. You can still continue to eat with your family and friends as long as you moderate your meals.

Planning your meals

Going on a diet entails not just changing one meal. It has to be done over a series of days, weeks, and even months. Obviously, you want to know what you should eat. To reverse the effects of diabetes and reduce blockages that may exist in the blood vessels and heart, you can refer to the following important tips.

1. Go for Unrefined Carbohydrates, Fruits, Vegetables

For the majority of your diet, you should prioritize these three groups. You're aiming for food that provides nutrition without the cholesterol, fats, or excessive sugar. Hence, these groups will serve to be your foundation towards healthier living.

Carbohydrates can affect your blood sugar levels. However, these are still essential for your bodily processes. In effect, you need to choose what kinds of food you should eat. Generally, you can go for unrefined carbohydrates. These are rich in fiber and are slow-release carbs. Slow-release carbs maintain your blood sugar as they take more time to be digested. Your body won't have to produce too much insulin and it would utilize the produced energy for longer periods of time. Moreover, you would feel full for a longer time. This would lessen your likelihood to crave for additional snacks. Some examples of excellent carb meals include: brown rice, low-sugar bran flakes, whole-wheat pasta, wheat bread, peas, and sweet potatoes.

The next set you should develop a liking for would be the vegetable group. In fact, all members of this group are considered healthy. What makes vegetables amazing is that they create their own food using photosynthesis. In effect, they can provide you a lot of energy for the day. Moreover, they are also rich in various vitamins. For example, green vegetables like broccoli, kale, and asparagus, are rich in iron and calcium. Orange vegetables like carrots, butternut squash, and yams have cancer fighting beta-carotene. As you can see, these don't only fight the effects of diabetes, but of other diseases as well. Having at least two or three vegetables on your dinner plate can go a long way. And if you think these aren't delicious, think again! Because these vegetables are natural and fresh, you can find these to be tasty additions to your meals. With the proper recipes, these can be a delight to your taste buds.

The vegetable group doesn't focus only on leafy greens. Legumes can be considered part of the group. Although people may overlook these, legumes can be promising. These include peas, lentils, and beans. Soy products like veggie burgers, tofu, miso, and other delights fall under this category also. What makes legumes amazing is that they are high in proteins that have low glycemic index (GI). Information on GI will be discussed in the next tip. They are also rich in iron, cholesterol-lowering soluble fiber, calcium, and even omega-3 fatty acids. It isn't surprising then that research has found that people who consume legumes regularly are thinner and healthier.

Fruits are the third group that you should love. Bursting with flavor, fruits pack a lot of vitamins for your body. More importantly, they contain no cholesterol or fat. Although some people are afraid to eat fruits because they are sweet, they don't raise your blood sugar. In fact, bananas, apples, blueberries, oranges, peaches, and almost all fruits have low GI. Pineapple and watermelon would be the exception. Because fruits are sweet, they can be used to create smoothies or afternoon snacks.

2. Look for food with low glycemic index (GI)

Glycemic index refers to how quickly food is transformed into sugar in your body. This analyzes the amount of carbohydrates and the glycemic index of a certain food. In other words, you will be able to know how a food can affect your blood sugar levels. High GI foods increase your blood sugar quickly, while low GI foods have minimal effects.

There are three groups that you can refer to as you monitor the GI. Fire foods are the ones to avoid; they have high GI and are low in protein and fiber. These include white foods like white pasta, white bread, sweets, and processed foods. Water foods are alright. You can eat as much as you like for these are healthy. These include fruits and vegetables. Coal foods are highly desirable. While these are high in protein and fiber, they have low GI. Nuts, seeds, whole grains, and beans are part of this category.

3. Supplement your meals with vitamins

Vitamins are necessary to boost your immune system and maintain a healthy body. While the mentioned food groups have got you covered, you should pay special attention to the vitamins that your body needs.

Calcium is important to maintain strong bones. Although people rely on milk to be the only source of calcium, beans and greens also provide plentiful amounts of the nutrient. Soy milk can also be an alternative option. However, while you increase calcium intake, you have to avoid factors that can reduce calcium in your body. Eating animal protein may lead to this risk as it lets calcium be removed through the kidneys. Sodium can also produce the same effects. Finally, to ensure that you do get the benefits of calcium, you should avoid harmful practices that may put you at risk for fractures or bone injuries. This includes smoking tobacco and engaging in extreme sports.

Vitamin B_{12} strengthens your blood cells and nerves. However you just need a small amount to gain the benefits of the vitamin. While this is found in fortified products, it is interesting to know that vitamin B_{12} is created by bacteria or other single-celled organisms. These organisms provide traces of the vitamin in the soil and it ends up in plants and animals. To satisfy your vitamin B_{12} needs, you can look for multivitamins in your local drug store.

Zinc boosts your immune system and assists in healing wounds. However, you have to keep this in moderation. Legumes, fortified cereals, and nuts are primary sources for zinc.

Vitamin D isn't something you eat. It's not even a vitamin. Rather, it is a hormone that is produced by sunlight when it interacts with your skin. It is converted to forms that pass through your kidneys and liver. In effect, Vitamin D helps you in absorbing calcium and strengthening your cells against cancer. To get Vitamin D, you just have to expose yourself to sunlight. While the process is simple, you have to do this in moderation. Overexposure may result in sunburn or to higher risks of skin cancer.

Iron can be both a boon and bane. As a boon, iron helps build hemoglobin. This would aid your bloodstream and oxygen regulation. However, too much iron can become toxic. In fact, high amounts can cause higher heart disease and insulin resistance risks. To ensure that your body gets safe levels of iron, you can consume green leafy vegetables and beans. Although these contain iron, the iron would be in the form called non-heme iron. In other words, the body would only absorb this form when it needs additional iron. If not, it can just leave your body through urination.

Chapter 5 - What to Avoid

Now that you know what to eat, you should also be aware about what foods to avoid. This doesn't mean completely removing these kinds of food in your life. Instead, you should monitor your intake of such food and minimize eating these. In controlling yourself when you eat these foods, you will be able to continue enjoying such food in the long run.

1. Minimize oil in general

Yes, vegetable oil can be better than animal fat. In fact, it can be found in salad oils, cooking oils, and vegetable oils for snacks and baking. However, although they may have less saturated fat, you should minimize all kinds of oil.

Whatever oil it may be, it will have much more calories than proteins or carbohydrates. The fat in oils have nine calories per gram, compared to four calories per gram in proteins or carbohydrates. This explains why oils and fats can be very fattening.

For some people, they might consider olive oil as an exception. However, you should realize that like other oils, this contains nine calories per gram. Since a lot of olives were processed to produce one bottle of oil, you shouldn't wonder why this provides a large amount of calories.

Since you also want to improve your sensitivity to insulin, you have to clean your body not only of animal fats but also of vegetable oils. As these carry grease, you have to refresh your body and flush those unwanted blockages away.

First, you should avoid fried foods. Potato chips, French fries, and all fried sponge-like snacks absorb grease and oil. These contribute to fat build-up in your body. Aside from these, you can avoid oils that are used as ingredients like sauces and packaged foods. Added oils found in salad dressings are also included in your "to avoid" list.

In case you find recipes that need oil for sautéing, you can execute these tips to create these dishes without using too much oil:

- Steam vegetables. You can also consider steam-frying garlic, onions, and other vegetables in water.

- Make use of nonstick pans.

- Use fat-free dressings for salads.

- Make sure to read the package labels and find products with less than two grams of fat per serving.

- Consider grilling, baking, broiling, or stir-frying.

Of course, vegetable oils can be naturally found in vegetables, beans, fruits, and grains. However, these shouldn't be alarming. Your body still needs a small amount of fat, and plants can provide these to you. If you do decide to use processed oils, you should use no more than five teaspoons in a day.

2. Lessen animal products

Eating less animal products boosts your health and increases weight loss. After all, you wouldn't be consuming fats from cows, chickens, and other meat sources. Because fats in muscle cells can rapidly increase if one is on a high-fat diet, you have to consider lessening or removing these kinds of food in your lifestyle.

Another major benefit you would get from avoiding animal products would involve removing the major source of cholesterol. You are guaranteed to improve your health significantly by avoiding these kinds of food and going for healthier options.

While you may be convinced that eating beef should be avoided, you may question whether you should avoid fish and chicken too. Well, chicken contains chicken fat. Even if the skin is removed, the white meat still contains 23% of its calories from fat. These fats would be saturated fat, a bad form of fat that increases your cholesterol. On the other hand, fish can have lower or higher fat content than chicken. However, whatever fish it may be, it will still have saturated fat. In fact, this would comprise around 20% of the fish fat. Hence, it can build up your cholesterol. Other seafood like lobsters and shrimps are worse alternatives as they are higher in cholesterol. Aside from meat, dairy products can contain high amounts of fat. A large amount of cow's milk calories (around 50%) comes from fat. Hence, foods like ice cream, yogurt, and sour cream products should be reduced.

Of course, while lessening your animal product intake can help, you don't have to permanently get rid of these. After all, they too have vital nutrients that your body needs for energy and muscle development. Hence, to moderate your intake, try eating a maximum of five ounces of protein every day. On the other hand, you can limit your dairy intake to three cups every day. However, if you can eat less of this prescribed amount, you will experience better effects. The key is in moderation.

3. Reduce sugar

As mentioned earlier, you don't have to live without sugar. Rather, you have to moderate your sugar intake so you can still enjoy your diet. Hence, you need to be smart in selecting when and what sweets to eat. Since sugar is located in many kinds of food like fast food, grocery store staples, and packaged meals, you need to be careful with what you buy. If you are able to cut sugar intake from these kinds of foods, you will have more room to eat sweet treats.

To determine if you should eat a certain food, you can check if it contains sugar. However, the ingredients list may hide sugar with other words to confuse you. Hence, you need to see if the ingredients list contains words that may be synonymous to sugar. These include: invert sugar, maltose, sugar, honey, agave nectar, corn sweetener, dextrose, evaporated cane juice, fructose, malt syrup, and many more.

To further cut down sugar, here are some added tips:

- Avoid packaged or processed foods. These include frozen dinners, low-fat meals, and other food that may have hidden sugar. Instead, try to prepare your own meals at home.

- Sweeten your own food. You can purchase plain yogurt, unsweetened iced tea, and other snacks, and use your own sweetener that can be made from fruits. This would be more refreshing and far healthier than artificial sweeteners.

- In preparing meals, reduce the amount of sugar. Instead of putting half a cup of sugar, you can put 1/3 cup of sugar. You can also choose to use natural sweeteners like nutmeg, cinnamon, and mint.

- Instead of eating the entire dessert, just eat half of it. To satisfy your cravings, you can replace the other half with fruits such as apples and oranges.

- Stick to water. Avoid drinking sugar-filled drinks like juice and soft drinks. According to research, drinking a 12 ounce serving of a sugar-sweetened beverage daily may increase your chances of diabetes by 15%. If you want to feel the sensation of carbonated drinks, you can try to drink sparkling water mixed with lemon. Furthermore, you can reduce the amount of sweeteners you use for tea and coffee.

Chapter 6 - Meal Tips and Suggestions

Having a healthy diet doesn't only refer to the meals you're supposed to eat. You have to consider your eating behavior. In completely adjusting your lifestyle to cater to your diabetes, you can improve your condition and minimize the effects of diabetes.

Meal Suggestions

Creating a healthy meal plan is challenging, yet fun. As much as possible, add variety to your meals so that you may appreciate them. You can also let your family eat these meals as these are nutritious and tasty. Below are some simple suggestions, however feel free to experiment on your own.

Breakfast

- Good Morning Mix: Get six ounces of fat-free yogurt, two tablespoons of ground flax seed, two tablespoons of dried mixed fruit, two tablespoons of chopped walnuts, almonds, or pecans, and two tablespoons of dried mixed fruit. Stir these together.

- Bagel delight: Spread a tablespoon of light cream cheese and a tablespoon of 100% fruit spread on half of a bagel (preferably whole grain).

- Oatmeal with a twist: Add ¼ cup of walnuts to half a cup of cooked oatmeal. You can opt to add cinnamon to create a sweeter taste.

- Vegetable omelet: Cook the egg in a pan with peanut or canola oil. Add half a cup of mushrooms, half a cup of spinach leaves, garlic, onions, and herbs. Place two tablespoons of reduced fat cheese on top.

- Assorted fruits: Create a mix using sliced bananas, apples, oranges, and mangoes.

Lunch

- Lean salad: Toss in two cups of mixed dark greens, an ounce of reduced-fat Mozzarella cheese, half a cup of canned garbanzo beans, and two tablespoons of light Italian dressing. Canned peaches can accompany this dish.

- Bean tostada: Using a 400-degree oven, bake one corn tortilla until it becomes crisp. Spread half a cup of cooked pinto beans and two tablespoons of reduced-fat cheese. Place the dish once more in the oven until the cheese melts. Serve with a cabbage salad.

- Pesto pizza: Get a 100% whole grain English muffin to be split and toasted. Afterwards, apply a tablespoon of pesto basil sauce, sliced tomatoes, and half a slice of low-fat cheese. Bake this until the cheese melts.

Dinner

- Stir fry tofu: Stir-fry three ounces of tofu and two cups of mixed vegetables (onions, broccoli, green beans, and cauliflower) in two tablespoons of stir fry sauce and a tablespoon of olive oil. Serve with brown rice.

- Cucumber salad: Toss a cup of cucumber slices, ten halved cheery tomatoes, a quarter of chopped red onions, two tablespoons of reduced-fat Italian dressing, and a cup of mixed greens. Serve with a fresh fruit smoothie.

- Mushroom Pasta: Toss a cup of cooked whole grain pasta in garlic. Add a tablespoon of olive oil. Add three ounces of mushrooms and a teaspoon of Parmesan cheese.

Snacks and Desserts

- Fresh fruit salad
- Mixed nuts
- Fruit shakes
- Sliced berries

Tips

Your body can control your blood sugar levels and weight if you practice a healthy meal schedule. For best results, you should eat consistent meal sizes. If you're overweight, you should remember that losing even just 7% of body weight can potentially cut the effects of diabetes by half. This can be done without having to deprive yourself of food!

Always eat breakfast. There's a reason why people say breakfast is the most important meal of the day. You will get your initial energy and nutrients from a hearty morning meal. If you don't eat breakfast, you may feel more fatigue and hungry for the rest of the day. In effect, you may overeat at lunch and dinner.

Eat small meals. One strategy some people use is to divide their three main meals into six smaller ones. These would be placed at regular intervals (6 am, 9 am, 12 pm, 3 pm, 6 pm, 9 pm). This can work in preventing you from overeating. Furthermore, your body will have a faster time metabolizing your food as this was consumed in smaller segments. Your risk of developing high blood sugar would decrease.

Maintain your calorie intake. To control your blood sugar, you can aim to eat a certain amount of calories per day. You can check the calorie counts of your meals and plan these strategically for you to avoid overeating or having to skip a meal.

Chapter 7 - Coping with the Real World

Although you have prepared meal plans and healthy recipes, you still have to face the food presented by the real world. While there are foods that are healthy and nutritious, it's obvious that there would also be food that may be too fatty, oily, or greasy. However, seeing how aesthetically pleasing these meals are, you may be tempted to give in and enjoy. Even if you can resist these kinds of food, there may be occasions when you simply can't refuse. In these moments, you shouldn't condemn yourself for entering such a situation. Instead, you can remember these tips to enjoy your eating experience while lessening the unwanted effects.

Fast Food

Almost everyone loves fast food. It can taste delicious and is very convenient for people in a hurry. However, fast foods have been associated with providing unhealthy food that may go against your diet plans. However, since these foods are delicious, you can create strategies to find ways to enjoy fast food. First of all, you can analyze the menus of these restaurants. Sure, there may be a multitude of fatty burgers and other meat-based meals. However, because fast food chains have been criticized for serving unhealthy food, many have attempted to create healthier menus. Salads and vegetable meals are growing trends in the fast food market.

Other than this, grilled burgers and healthier meals have been prepared for the enjoyment of their consumers. With these new additions, you can choose to consume these options. Of course, if you do choose to eat a greasy burger, you should consider the implications of these meals. If you could easily exercise and burn the gained calories, then you shouldn't have much problem eating these in moderation. You just have to prepare to work hard to recover from the consequences of eating such food.

Dining Out

Not all restaurants serve fast food. There are fancy or humble restaurants that prepare meals of varying flavors. People want to dine out not only to enjoy the food, but to get together with their friends, family, and loved ones. As dining with others can bring joy and release stress, you shouldn't worry over such occasions. Be smart and choose healthy options.

In selecting a restaurant, you should remember that international cuisine may be healthier. As Asian, Latin American, and Mediterranean countries have traditional staples such as rice, legumes, vegetables, fruits, and grains, these can be ideal choices. It isn't surprising that these regions have lower diabetes rates compared to those in Western Europe and North America.

An example would be Italian cuisine. Italian restaurants are home to salads, grilled vegetable pizzas, steamed spinach, pasta, and other delectably healthy meals. For better food, you can request the chef to avoid adding cheese and lessen oil usage. If you're craving for Asian flavors, you can also consider Chinese restaurants. These are famous for steamed spring rolls, healthy soups, and vegetables. It is best to pick steamed food over fried meals. Instead of getting meat dishes, you can explore the vegetable and tofu menu. While these kinds of meals are delectable, it is possible that more oil is used to prepare these. Hence, you may advise the chef to reduce the oil. Other than this, you can also request to use brown rice instead of white rice.

Vietnamese and Thai restaurants may serve more nutritious foods that are mainly steamed. Hence, you should utilize their vegetable meals, rice, noodles, and tofu. Perhaps one of the best Asian cuisines would be Japanese food. This includes healthy sushi that is created from rice, cucumber, mango, and other fruits and vegetables. They also serve seaweed, salads, and miso soup. On the other hand, if you are craving spicy dishes, you can try out Latin American cuisine. The menu is rich in salads, salsa, black bean dishes, and other similar food.

Of course, for an enjoyable and healthy experience, you shouldn't be afraid to make special requests. Speaking up to ask for the removal of bacon flakes, cheese, and other unwanted ingredients is the key to being responsible with one's diet. Usually, these restaurants permit the changes and would immediately comply with their customer's requests. This doesn't mean the meal will be less sumptuous. They will find alternative ways to improve the dish without using those ingredients. Hence, the individual will have a better meal and help the restaurant as it is exposed to different kinds of patrons. Furthermore, to be on the safe side, you can also ask how the food is prepared. This would be useful to see if they use too much oil or other unwanted condiments.

Attending special occasions

There will be instances when you will get invited to parties, anniversaries, and wedding celebrations. Of course, it would be rude to avoid these events, especially if these were organized by people close to you. However, it would be unwise to eat all of the undesired food while you are there. Hence, you must plan before attending the event so that you can enjoy without sacrificing your healthy practices.

First, perhaps the best way to prepare is to eat a meal before going to the occasion. By the time you arrive, you wouldn't feel that hungry. In effect, you would be there to eat some light food and avoid consuming large amounts of food that goes against your meal plan. Instead, you can focus more on talking with the other guests and enjoying the program.

You can also bring a healthy meal. If you were invited for lunch or dinner, you wouldn't know what will be served. In these cases, you can call the hosts and honestly explain to them your situation. Afterwards, you can offer to bring food like a fresh fruit salad or vegetable soup. Assuming that the host is on good terms with you, they would warmly accept your offer. Often times, they may even say that there is no need to bring additional food as they would provide alternatives to cater to your needs. People are generally very accepting and encouraging if you tell them that you are eating differently because of diabetes, or simply because you're trying to improve your health.

Another suggestion for parties is to have a plate. When moving around a party, you can carry a plate with some bread, fruits, or vegetables. Going around empty-handed may be a sign for others to offer the diabetic food. To avoid these awkward situations, it is best to have something on hand. This would also make it easier to refuse any offers as you may explain that you are already full.

If you are offered something you don't desire, politely refuse. You don't need to make a big deal out of the offer. Calmly refusing the food is a better choice than being pressured to eat it and regretting your choices after. As an independent individual, you should know what your limits are, and let people understand that these should be respected.

Finally, you should still have fun during the party. Stress is a negative reaction that can contribute not only to diabetes, but to other health conditions. Hence, while you may stress over food choices, this shouldn't engulf you to the point wherein you are no longer enjoying the party.

Traveling

Food is abundant when you travel. As you visit different cities and countries, you may want to immerse yourself in different cultures. This includes the local cuisine and delicacies. Since you would be following a diet, you have to wisely choose which restaurants to eat in. Most places have vegan and non-vegan restaurants. Others would offer fast food or fine dining restaurants. It would all depend on the location. For best results, you can try to search the internet regarding food locations in the area you're visiting. From there, you can plan in advance all the restaurants you would like to visit and what to order. This will save you time and cause you less stress when you get to your destination.

Since traveling on plane can last for several hours, you can also request for a vegan meal before the flight. In effect, the crew will serve you a healthier meal and require no additional charges. For short domestic flights, you can try to bring your own snacks. Vegan sandwiches, soy milk, baby carrots, or other snacks wouldn't be a problem on these trips. If you aren't able to bring any food, you can ask the flight attendants if fruits are available.

Drinking Alcohol

If you like drinking alcohol, you may wonder if you will have to give this up to maintain your diet. Luckily, having diabetes shouldn't be a reason for you to stop drinking. In fact, as long as you can maintain your blood sugar level, you can drink alcohol in moderation. Alcohol can be useful in reducing your risk for heart disease. Ideally, men should drink no more than 2 drinks a day while women should drink no more than one. One drink is equivalent to five ounces of wine, twelve ounces of beer, or one and a half ounces of distilled spirits. Furthermore, before drinking, you can try asking yourself these questions:

- Is my diabetes under control?

- Do I have health problems that can worsen because of alcohol intake?

- Do I know how drinking alcohol can affect me?

Alcohol can move quickly within your bloodstream without being metabolized within the stomach. In fact, after five minutes, your bloodstream can contain a significant amount of alcohol. This would be metabolized by the liver. Usually, it takes two hours for a drink to be metabolized. Alcohol can be dangerous if you're taking insulin or other diabetes medications because it can stimulate your pancreas to create more insulin. In effect, you may develop low blood sugar or hypoglycemia because your liver would have to work harder to get rid of the alcohol. It would be diverted to this task instead of regulating your blood sugar.

To ensure that you remain healthy while drinking alcohol, you should practice drinking with caution. Avoid drinking on an empty stomach or if your blood sugar is low. To be safe, drink while eating food. Alongside your alcohol, you can also have a zero calorie beverage like water or iced tea.

You should also take your time when drinking. Sip slowly and make your drink last. This helps your body metabolize the alcohol much better.

Furthermore, you shouldn't be ashamed to make your drinking buddies aware that you are diabetic. Always bring glucose tabs or other sugar sources to prevent low blood sugar. You can also opt to wear an ID that explains that you have diabetes. Since alcohol may cause hypoglycemia, which can show similar symptoms to being drunk, it is best that people are aware of your condition so that they take you seriously if you do suffer from hypoglycemia.

Eating with the family

While you may be excited to try out your new diet, your family might not be. Instead, they may insist on eating lots of meat or other meals that don't fit anywhere in your meal plans. In these cases, you may try to fix healthy meals for yourself and less healthy meals for your family. Of course, the better option is to slowly introduce to them the benefits of healthy food. Moreover, you should try to convince them that healthy food can be delicious. Hence, an ideal situation involves the entire family agreeing to change their diet. If everyone is aware of the benefits, it is possible for them to agree with whatever changes you want to implement. These discussions should be approached with love. If ever your family members refuse, respect their decision. Do not force them to agree to your proposal. However, make sure that they do know why you are making such a change so that they too may realize how alarming diabetes can be.

If ever they do agree, don't rush the sudden meal changes. Do it slowly. As they learn to adjust to the food, they will slowly get used to the meals.

Chapter 8 - Additional Advice

In the previous chapters, you were exposed to tips and techniques on how to improve your diet to fight diabetes. While these tackle the principles on proper food planning and behavior, sometimes, you may feel that nothing is happening. Your weight may still be the same, or it may still continue increasing. During these moments, you shouldn't fear. Rather, you can refer to these reminders.

No Weight Loss? No problem!

You shouldn't worry if you aren't losing weight in the first few days of the diet. Your plans are set for long-term purposes. You're not starving yourself to immediately lose pounds. However, if you feel that nothing has changed after several weeks, you can start reassessing your diet. First, you can go back to the basics. You can refer to the principles discussed in the previous chapters and step up your game. For example, if you still eat a minimal amount of meat products, you can further reduce that and increase your vegetable and fruit intake.

You can also simplify your meals. Instead of using processed foods, you can use fewer ingredients. Just focus on vegetables and legumes for your meals instead of creating sauces or other additions for your dish. As there may be hidden oils in added ingredients, you have to remain cautious.

On the other hand, you can also try using more raw food. To decrease oil intake, you can just chop vegetables or prepare salads. These will be richer in fiber without having to worry about high GIs and extra fat.

In addition to these improvements, you should remember that a food diary is your friend. Studies have shown that individuals who keep food diaries lose more weight. Why? Apparently, they are more aware of what they eat. They can identify problems in their diets and create alternatives to resolve these. Because of their increased awareness, they on average lose twice as much compared to those who don't keep a diary.

Can't control blood glucose?

To see your progress in terms of blood sugar levels, you will have to undergo the same test you used to detect diabetes. Here, you will find an accurate reading of your blood glucose levels over the course of your diet. Most clinicians would want your hemoglobin A1c test to read a result of under 6.5 %. If you haven't reached that goal, you can consider improving your diet.

First, you have to love healthy carbohydrates. If you feel worried that beans, rice, or other starchy vegetables are causing your blood sugar levels to rise, shrug off the feeling. These are better options than going back to full meat meals. Some people make the mistake of leaving their diets and returning to meat-based meals. However, although they may initially think that their blood sugar levels are going down, these will gradually rise and eventually reach a significantly high level. Always remember that carbohydrates, proteins, and fat are the three sources of calories. If you shun the carbohydrates group, you will only have protein foods, which cause insulin resistance, and fatty foods, which may increase cholesterol. Compared to carbohydrates, these food types lead to bigger spikes in your blood sugar.

If you still have difficulty controlling your blood glucose, you can go to your doctor. Infections can also cause rising blood sugar. Colds, foot sores, urinary tract infections, and other sicknesses may be causing you discomfort. Hence, your doctor can help you detect if your blood sugar levels are caused by your diet or something else.

Always feeling hungry? Don't be!

Going on a diet doesn't equate to starving yourself. Although you'll eat lower amounts of certain foods, you shouldn't eat less in general. In fact, you have to eat more if you feel hungry. For example, if you still feel hungry even after eating a bowl of oatmeal, you can try to add more oatmeal. You just have to figure out the right serving sizes that will satisfy your hunger.

You can also focus more on high fiber and low GI meals. Eating natural food will prevent rapid digestion that leaves you hungry. Other than this, you should still be able to maintain your blood sugar and perform well. If you do continue to be hungry, you can try to eat more healthy snacks. Fresh fruits are excellent choices.

Other Reminders

Eating right isn't enough to make your diet work. You have to accompany this with other lifestyle changes.

> **Exercise.** Eating isn't your only concern. To maximize the results, you have to exercise to help your body burn fat and remain healthy. Research has shown that insulin sensitivity can be improved through regular exercise. You don't have to spend hours in the gym to exercise. Walking, playing sports, or other physical activities are sufficient for your bodily needs. What's important is that you find the

time to move, even for just thirty minutes, to remain fit. Here are some kinds of exercises you can do to help your well-being:

- Resistance exercise revolves around weight lifting and similar activities which works on your muscles. These include pushups and pull-ups. In building your muscle mass, you would preserve the muscles you have and avoid muscle atrophy. Resistance exercises can also improve your insulin sensitivity.

- Flexibility exercises involve stretching which helps maintain your joint motion. Because this can relieve stress, you will be able to function better and maintain lower levels of blood sugar.

- Aerobic exercises are popular and fun. These use continuous and rhythmic activities that last around ten minutes. Here, you will dance, walk, run, skate, or play sports. This would be beneficial in reducing your triglycerides and blood sugar.

Sleeping habits. It is best for you to maintain at least 8 hours of sleep every day. This helps the body recuperate from a long day and gives it time to break down all of the food you've eaten. Proper sleep will also release natural hormones that can improve your bodily processes. Furthermore, if you wake up refreshed, you will be able to work better and feel less tired. This is important to prevent yourself from overeating to overcome feelings of fatigue.

About stress. You should find activities to release your stress and minimize this. Stress can build negative hormones in your body and cause complications to arise. This will also make your body work more and can raise your blood sugar levels. Although temporary stress will result in temporary glucose spikes, continuous stress should be attended to. You can try to watch movies, listen to music, meditate, or do yoga. While maintaining your busy lifestyle, you have to make room for fun and relaxation.

Attitude. Remembering that dieting is a long-term process, you have to maintain the right attitude. If ever you don't meet your expectations and set goals, don't fret. You shouldn't be disheartened. Continue working. At least you've made attempts to control your diabetes. Having a fighting attitude is important if you want to reduce the effects of your condition. If ever you feel down, don't let it grow on you. Instead, you can readjust your priorities and see where you may be lacking. From there, you can continue to improve. Whatever happens, don't give up.

By now, you should realize that you have the capacity to control your diabetes. This monster may be overwhelming, but with the proper techniques, food, and mindset, you can surpass this difficulty and continue on with your life. In following these simple tips, you can definitely live life to the fullest instead of letting diabetes control you. Of course, you don't have to do this by yourself. You can encourage friends and loved ones to try out these tips. After all, these tips aren't only concerned for people with diabetes, but for everyone who wants to live healthier and better.

Conclusion

Thank you again for downloading this book!

I hope this book was able to help you learn more about improving diabetes with diet and lifestyle choices.

The next step is to take action and put the strategies in this book into use! And of course, always remember to consult a medical professional when starting a diet or exercise program for their guidance.

Finally, if you enjoyed this book, please take the time to share your thoughts and post a review on Amazon. It'd be greatly appreciated!

Thank you and good luck!

www.ingramcontent.com/pod-product-compliance
Lightning Source LLC
LaVergne TN
LVHW021740060526
838200LV00052B/3386